To María Pilar, Emilios and Carlos.

To Nacho, Violeta and Marcos.

The author

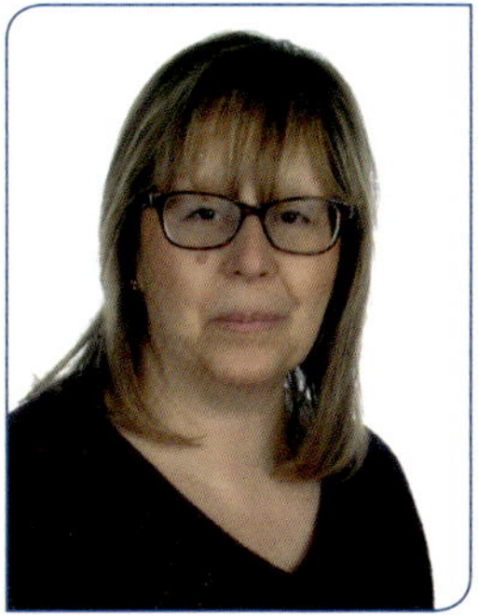

María Victoria Falceto Recio

DVM, MS, PhD

Permanent lecturer in Reproduction and Obstetrics, Department of Animal Pathology, Faculty of Veterinary Medicine, University of Zaragoza, Zaragoza, Spain.

AI and Hormone Management in the Sow

1 AI in pigs: current approach

Artificial insemination (AI) is a routine procedure on commercial pig farms worldwide. This method of **assisted reproduction** replaces natural mating to achieve pregnancy by depositing semen in the sow's reproductive tract using a catheter.

AI makes work on the farm easier and minimises transmission of sexual diseases, but only a small number of sows can be inseminated in the productive lifetime of the boar. Currently, the number of sperm needed for a semen AI dose is reducing, and hormone management reduces the number of inseminations to a single session. This allows insemination of a single sow or even of a group of sows with semen from a single boar, and hence genetic improvement (only the best boars are used). Future research will also facilitate artificial insemination with frozen and/or sexed semen on commercial farms.

Routine semen evaluation at pig AI centres (AICs) is very comprehensive, and any poor quality ejaculate is discarded. Many AICs use precise and repeatable methods to analyse the semen, using computer programs that evaluate individual sperm. This enables them to produce more semen AI doses per ejaculate, using fewer sperm but retaining a very high quality.

Despite the rigorous semen analysis provided by computer-assisted sperm analysis systems, the use of certain boars can still lead to poor fertility and prolificacy on some farms. Some laboratories offer testing to evaluate the fertilisation potential (in vitro fertilisation tests) and sperm characteristics that determine the viability of the embryo after fertilisation (flow cytometry, etc.). In the future, before young boars with high genetic value are admitted to an AIC, they will be submitted to these tests, with additional cytogenetic studies to detect chromosome abnormalities.

The minimum AIC values for semen quality are: more than 70 % motility, less than 25–30 % morphological abnormalities and more than 80 % intact acrosomes.

Oestrous cycle

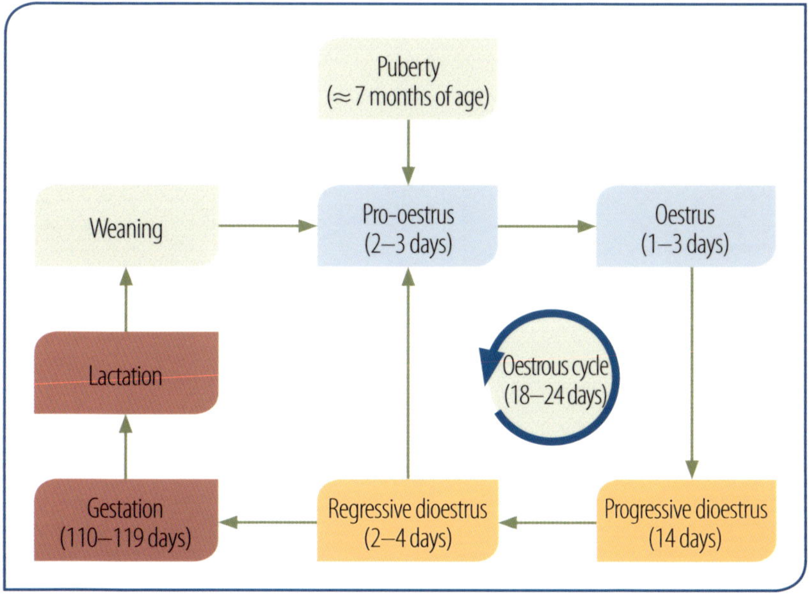

Figure 1. The reproductive cycle in the sow. Oestrous cycle: Follicular phase (4–6 days) shown in blue and luteal phase (16–18 days) shown in orange.

Signs of oestrus

Oestrogens (E2) are the most important hormones produced during the follicular phase and they cause visible signs of oestrus in the sow. These signs are as follows:

Changes in normal sow behaviour

- Loss of appetite.
- Characteristic grunting.
- Restlessness and increased activity.
- Biting the bars and feeders.
- Increased movement around the pen.
- Standing to be mounted, or increased tendency to mount other sows.
- Arched back.
- **Standing reflex** when pressure is applied to her back.

Changes in sow behaviour in the presence of a teaser boar

- Searching for the boar.
- Ears pricked.
- Frequent urination.
- Salivation.
- **Standing reflex** in the presence of the boar.

Characteristics of the genitalia

- Tail raised and twitching, exposing the vulva.
- Vulva swollen and reddened.
- Mucus secreted from vulva.

Not all sows show all the signs listed. The sow's standing reflex in the presence of the boar is an unmistakable sign of oestrus.

Detection of oestrus

Detection of oestrus and artificial insemination are two distinct tasks on the farm. Detection of oestrus aims to identify the start and end of oestrus in each sow, so that insemination can be scheduled according to the procedures in place on that particular farm. A much higher percentage of sows in heat will be detected if observation for signs of oestrus are rigorous. **Physical contact between the sow and a boar will maximise effective detection of oestrus.** The sow exhibits oestrus most clearly when she can see, hear, smell, and touch a boar, which makes identification easier for the person in charge of detecting oestrus.

Some farms make the mistake of detecting oestrus without the presence of a boar. Only 50 % of sows in oestrus react with the standing reflex to pressure exerted on the back by a person. Oestrous behaviour in the sow can be increased to 70 % by the use of pheromone sprays, and using a boar increases this figure to almost 100 %.

Choice of staff and boar

Detection of oestrus should be performed by designated farm staff using teaser boars.

The designated staff should have **specific training** and be aware of the consequences of doing their job poorly. In hot weather, oestrus can be less obvious so detection of oestrus should be assigned to the best trained member of farm staff.

Teaser boars should be **tractable** and have a high **libido**. Every farm should have several teaser boars so that they can be used in rotation. Teaser boars can be entire, epidectomised or vasectomised, and they should be allowed to mate with culled sows to maintain their libido.

Boars are also used to stimulate sows sexually to bring on oestrus (boar effect) and to increase uterine contractions during intracervical insemination.

Frequency of detection of oestrus

Detection of oestrus should be carried out **at least once a day**. A protocol to detect oestrus should comprise one or two sessions per day. A sow in oestrus will only be receptive to the boar for 10–15 minutes after first seeing him. She will then get used to him and can stop exhibiting oestrous behaviour for almost an hour.

Sows requiring detection of oestrus

The protocol should include **all sows** on the farm that are not pregnant:

- Gilts >6 months of age.
- Postweaning sows.
- Inseminated sows that have not yet been confirmed as pregnant.
- Sows diagnosed as not pregnant.
- Sows in anoestrus.

Although gilts are not inseminated until their third oestrus, ensure that their first and second oestrus are recorded.

It is usually advisable to carry out the detection procedure twice a day.

Also sows that are suspected of being in oestrus, despite already being in the pregnant sow group.

Methods for oestrus detection

Detection of oestrus in pens

There is very close contact between the boar and sow. The boar will sniff the sow's genitals, nose, and carpal joints, put his head under her belly and nudge her flanks with the top of his snout, while making small grunting noises. Finally, he may put his chin on the sow's hindquarters and attempt to mount. The sow in oestrus will remain totally still during this courtship phase. Once identified, the sow should be marked and removed so that the boar can continue teasing with the other sows in the group. There should be no more than three sows in a group, to avoid intimidating the boar. Two or three boars that have been raised together should be used at the same time to test bigger groups.

Farm design can make effective detection of oestrus either easier or more difficult. The boar can only perform the courtship ritual to the extent that the available facilities on the farm allow.

The boar sniffs the carpal sweat glands because they secrete pheromones.

Detection of oestrus in crates

The boar walks up the passage in front of the crates. A system of gates is advisable, allowing each boar to be presented to 4–5 sows for 5–10 minutes at a time. If facilities permit, more sows can be tested at the same time using several boars that have been raised together. On some farms, the boar is controlled by a harness or moved along inside a mobile crate, sometimes with remote control. The boar will sniff the sow's face and carpal joints. The sow will see, hear, and smell the boar and become immobile if she is in oestrus. At the same time, another worker should move along behind the crates, massaging sows' flanks and pressing on their back to confirm oestrus (sows can allow themselves to be sat on without them moving).

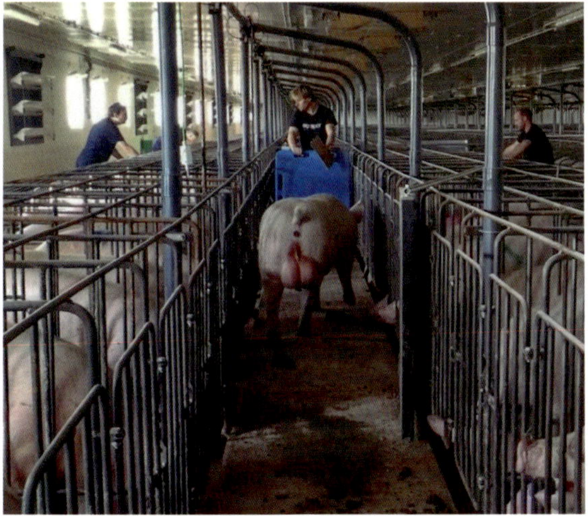

Figure 2. Boar in the passage. System of gates that allows management of oestrus detection.

Consequences of poor oestrus detection

If the person assigned to detection fails to detect any signs, even though the sow is in oestrus, she will be marked as an anoestrous sow, although she is actually in pseudoanoestrus. As the sow is already in oestrus, she cannot respond to hormone treatments to induce oestrus and is usually wrongly removed from the farm.

Sometimes, ineffective detection of oestrus can lead to sows being inseminated too early or too late in relation to ovulation. These animals either do not conceive or give birth to small litters.

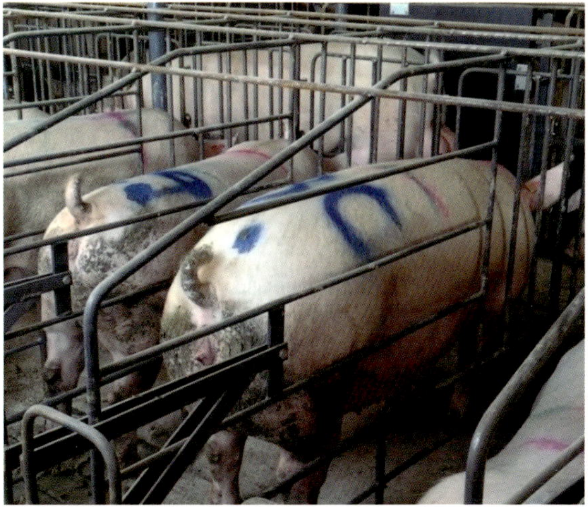

Figure 3. The number of people assigned to detection of oestrus should be sufficient to confirm the detection by the boar and mark these sows.

The fertilisation process requires the sperm and oocyte to meet in the ampulla of the oviduct at a particular moment in their lifespan. Oocytes are viable for about eight hours after ovulation. Sperm have fertilisation potential in the reproductive tract for approximately 24 hours after insemination, but they do require about six hours to fully mature (capacitation) before they are able to fertilise.

If the sperm or oocyte is aged, the sow will probably not conceive, or embryo survival and litter size will be reduced. It is very important to identify the best moment for artificial insemination during oestrus for each sow to reduce reproductive failure on the farm.

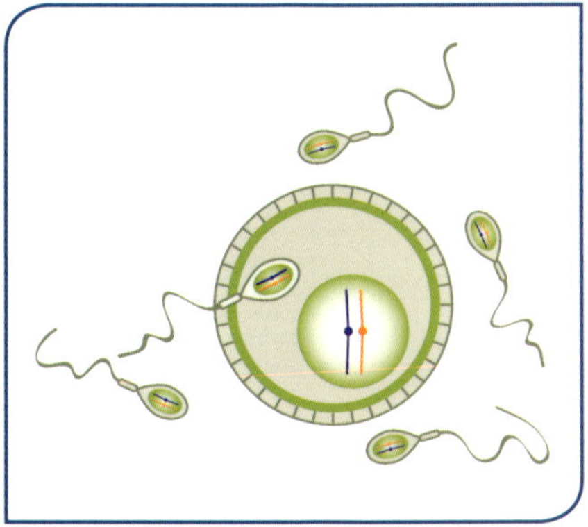

Figure 1. Fertilisation.

When to inseminate

Artificial insemination should take place **close to ovulation** to ensure fertilisation and maximise litter size.

During oestrus, the sow does not display any visible signs that ovulation has occurred. As the moment of ovulation is unknown, a sow in oestrus would need to be inseminated several times at intervals of 12–24 hours in order for fertile sperm to always be waiting in the oviduct when ovulation takes place. This necessitates a great deal of work for the farm and demands trained personnel. It also increases the risk of uterine infections and requires more semen doses and insemination equipment.

There is currently a trend for pig farms to try to reduce the number of inseminations per sow in oestrus. If the precise moment of ovulation was known, the sow would only have to be inseminated once during the preceding 8–12 hours.

Insemination based on estimating the moment of ovulation

Despite research into many methods of detecting the moment of ovulation, there is still no truly effective, cheap method that is easy for farm personnel to use. The techniques investigated so far are based on changes in various parameters during oestrus: luteinising hormone (LH) levels, temperature of the vulva, vaginal cytology, electrical resistance of the vaginal mucus, etc. Diagnosis by ultrasound examination of the ovary is extremely precise, but it requires highly skilled personnel and lengthy evaluation. The most common technique currently used by farms to estimate the moment of ovulation (AI) is based on the determination of the onset and end of oestrus.

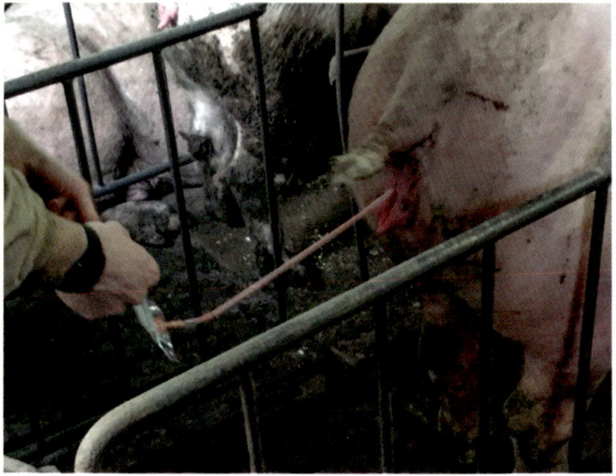

Figure 2. Insemination and the standing reflex in the sow.

Duration of oestrus

Oestrus starts with the appearance of the **standing reflex** in the sow and ends when is ceases. It lasts approximately two days (between one and five days). **Ovulation** occurs **70 % of the way through oestrus** (Kirkwood and Kauffold, 2015).

The main problem when estimating the interval between the start of oestrus and ovulation is that the end of the standing reflex is unknown. The duration of oestrus and the moment of ovulation also vary significantly between sows. This variability depends on the following factors:

- Genetics.
- Age: gilts or multiparous sows.
- Start of oestrus after weaning.
- Time of year.
- Farm: temperature, humidity, ventilation, lighting, welfare, stress, nutrition, lactation length, 'boar effect', protocol for detection of oestrus, etc.

Every farm should record the start and end of oestrus in their sows and calculate the average **duration** (Table 1). However, this information can be **subjective**, as it depends on operator training and the method and frequency of detection of oestrus on the farm.

Table 1. Average duration of oestrus (hours) in multiparous sows.

Week of the year	Average	Range	Week of the year	Average	Range
1	56.2	(42–72)	6	55.2	(42–72)
2	59.4	(36–84)	7	62.1	(36–84)
3	60.4	(36–72)	8	56.2	(36–72)
4	54.7	(36–84)	9	61.3	(36–84)
5	63.6	(36–72)	10	61.5	(48–72)
			Overall farm average	**59.06 (n=400)**	**(36–84)**

Effect of age on the duration of oestrus and the timing of insemination

Oestrus is very short in some **gilts** and ovulation can occur on the first day, so insemination is recommended as soon as the standing reflex is seen. The gilt should be inseminated again 24 hours later. This behaviour is caused by immaturity of the hypothalamic–pituitary–ovarian axis related to age.

The duration of oestrus in **multiparous sows** is very variable. Hypothalamic–pituitary–ovarian axis functioning in these sows is related to the lactation period that has just ended. Recommendations for inseminating postweaning females mainly depend on the interval between weaning and oestrus (Table 2).

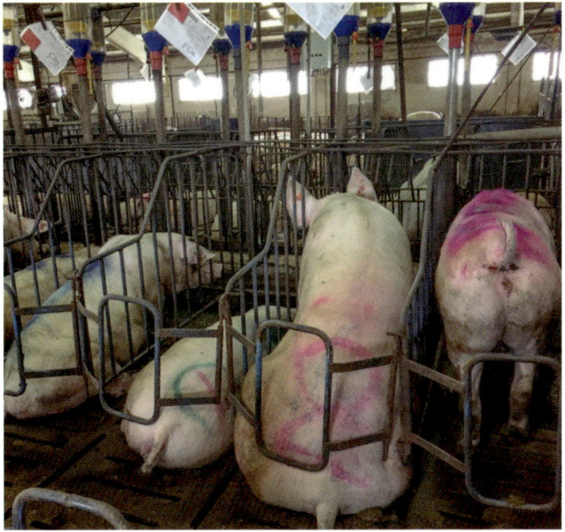

Figure 3. The duration of oestrus varies between sows, depending on the interval between weaning and oestrus.

Effect of weaning-to-oestrus interval (WOI) on the duration of oestrus and timing of insemination

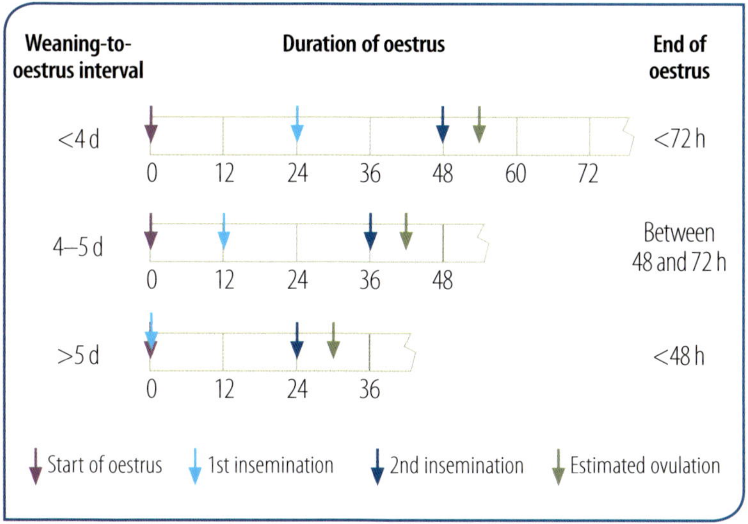

If the sow has returned to oestrus or aborted, it is advisable to inseminate as soon as oestrus is detected and again 24 hours later.

Figure 4. Estimation of the moment of ovulation, and insemination protocol. The interval between the 1st and 2nd AI is always 24 hours. The longer the WOI, the shorter the oestrus and the more the ovulation is brought forward.

Measuring luteinising hormone (LH)

Luteinising hormone can be measured on-farm with a commercial kit. The problem with monitoring LH is that it requires blood or urine to be taken at least every six hours from the start of oestrus until the LH reaches a peak (5–7 ng/ml) prior to ovulation. As this peak is very short-lived, it may not be detected if sampling is carried out at longer intervals.

Temperature of the vulva

Reddening of the vulva due to the increased blood flow to the sow's reproductive tract is related to the increase in oestrogen levels during the follicular phase. These oestrogen levels will reach a peak, and then oestradiol will decrease until ovulation occurs. It appears that the temperature of the skin of the vulva during oestrus may parallel the reddening of the vulva, though this has been questioned. Changes in vulval temperature (°C) can be measured with an infrared thermometer or thermal imaging camera. The main problem with these methods is that the temperature of the vulva can be affected by many factors that are not related to follicular dynamics or the actual ovulation process.

Vaginal cytology

Diagnosis by vaginal cytology is based on changes in the thickness of the stratified squamous epithelium of the sow's vagina throughout the oestrous cycle. The number of layers in the epithelium reaches its maximum following the oestrogen peak before the preovulatory LH surge. An increase in superficial cells found by vaginal smear indicates the sow is in oestrus. This technique is very widely used in other species (such as the dog) due to its high predictive value. However, this is very low in the sow, and it also requires trained personnel.

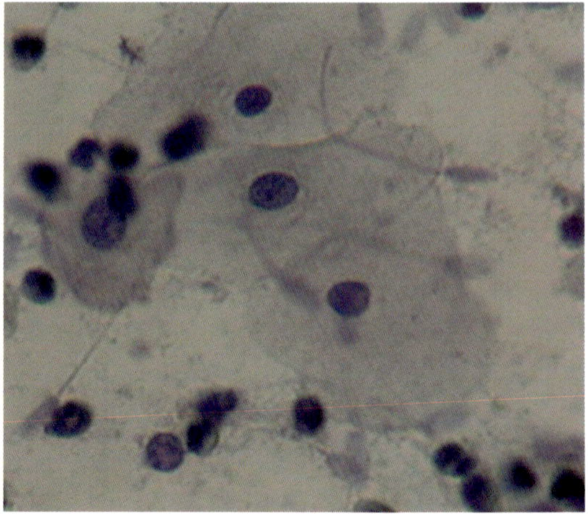

Figure 5. Superficial cells predominate on a vaginal smear from a sow in oestrus. Sperm remain from insemination before the sample was taken.

Electrical resistance of the vaginal mucus

Changes in the electrical resistance of the vaginal mucus (measured in ohms) are monitored using a galvanometer. These are measured inside the vagina, so equipment must be cleaned and disinfected between sows to prevent cross-infection. A gradual reduction can be detected in the electrical resistance of the vaginal mucus linked to increasing oestrogen levels. This is followed by an increase before ovulation. However, no practical test has yet been established that can be used on pig farms to determine the moment of ovulation in individual sows.

Ultrasound is useful in confirming whether or not the usual protocol for AI used on a specific pig farm is adequate with respect to determining the moment of ovulation.

Ultrasound examination of the ovary

Growth of the ovarian follicles is monitored every six hours from the start of oestrus until the follicles reach preovulatory size. Ovulation is detected when the large follicles (>6.5 mm) disappear from the ovary and the corpora rubra appear.

Modern **abdominal ultrasound** equipment allows the moment of ovulation to be detected on commercial farms. The cost of ultrasound equipment and the requirement for highly trained personnel are disadvantages that can be overcome by assigning this procedure to consultant veterinary specialists.

Fixed-time artificial insemination

Using hormones to induce and synchronise ovulation

Inducing and synchronising ovulation with hormones allows the interval between hormone administration and ovulation to be predicted, enabling insemination to be carried out 10–12 hours before ovulation. The sperm undergo capacitation in this time, and are ready to fertilise the oocytes immediately after their release at ovulation. Porcine LH, hCG, , and GnRH analogues can be used: buserelin, gonadorelin, goserelin, lecirelin, peforelin, triptorelin, etc. Each hormone has its own protocol for use.

Use of encapsulated semen

One single insemination with encapsulated semen ensures that there are viable male gametes in the oviduct at ovulation. The sperm are held in a matrix and their cellular structure and functionality are maintained during storage (15 °C). After insemination, the sperm (38 °C) are gradually released over a longer period of time. The capsule protects against semen backflow from the vulva and uterine phagocytosis, and prevents premature spermatozoa capacitation (Sánchez et al., 2014). This technique requires further investigation before being used on commercial farms.

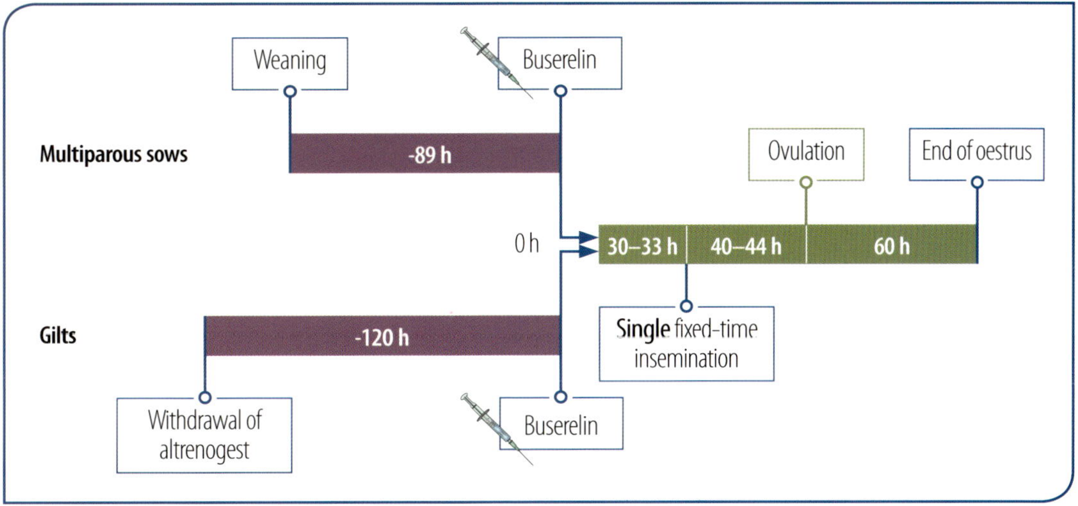

Figure 6. Ovulation induction in gilts and multiparous sows, using fixed-time insemination.

When to stop inseminating

Insemination should cease when the sow stops displaying a standing reflex. Some farms employ a third or fourth forced late insemination. In some cases, if oestrus has been detected too late, the second insemination may be a forced one, which is equally unnecessary.

Bacteria can enter with the semen during insemination but when the sow is in oestrus, oestrogens strengthen local defences in the uterus and these can eliminate the bacteria. However, bacteria multiply easily in the uterus after **late insemination**, as the progesterone in the luteal phase tends to reduce local defences in the uterus to prevent the paternal antigens in the embryo from being rejected in the event of conception. Progesterone also reduces uterine contractions, increasing secretions in the lumen of the uterus.

Because the cervix closes during dioestrus, a sow with **postinsemination endometritis** will not display a vulvar discharge. It is not until the opening of the cervix at the start of the next follicular phase that any secretions are able to escape. This is during pro-oestrus, just before the sow returns to oestrus.

A sow with a vulvar discharge should never be inseminated.

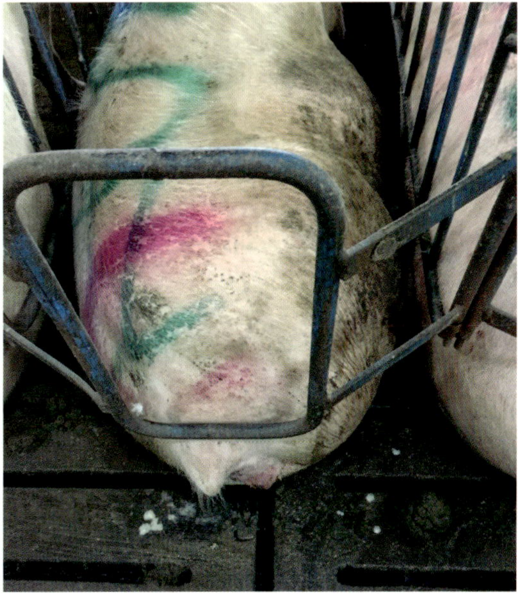

Figure 7. Vulval discharge syndrome: purulent discharge.

Preparation of the semen

Microscopic evaluation of the semen before artificial insemination

The causes of infertility are equally shared between the boar and the sow. On arrival at the farm, it is essential to assess the **sperm motility** of the dose immediately before insemination to verify that it has not been affected by temperature changes during transport or by semen preservation methods. The steps to follow are:

Step 1. Turn on the external warming plate or the microscope stage warmer. When the temperature reaches 38 °C, place the slide and coverslip on the warmer to come up to temperature (Fig. 1).

Caution! Temperatures <37 °C do not allow **true sperm motility** to be assessed and >39 °C can **kill the sperm.**

Step 2. Remove a dose for each boar from which semen will be used that day for AI on the farm from the semen storage unit (15–17 °C). Warm the doses in a water bath at 37 °C.

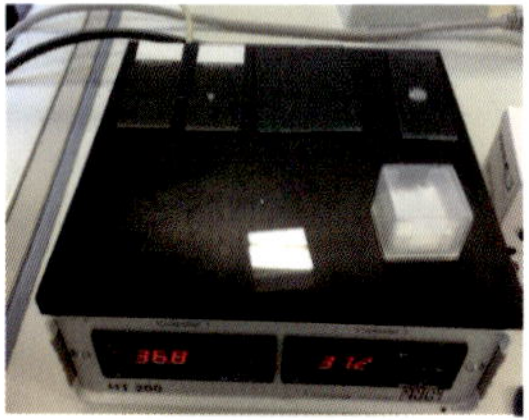

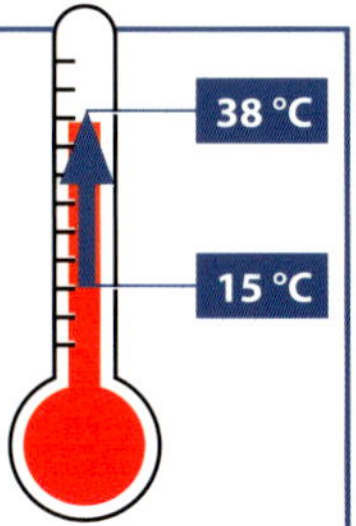

Figure 1. Warming plate (left). The thermometer shows the difference between the storage temperature and the correct temperature to evaluate motility (right).

Step 3. Check that the dose has not passed its expiry date.

Step 4. Gently rotate 2–3 times to mix the contents (Fig. 2).

Step 5. Using a Pasteur pipette, place one drop of semen on the slide and cover it with the coverslip, both already at a temperature of 38 °C. **The drop should be big enough to fill the coverslip area so that no air bubbles remain to make observation difficult.**

Step 6. Assess the sample with a light microscope:

- View at 100, 200 and 400 times magnification (10× eyepiece and 10×, 20× and 40× objectives).
- Obtain the percentage of sperm with motility (0–100 %) by counting at least 4 different optical fields.
- Do not include sperm that are clumped together (Fig. 3).

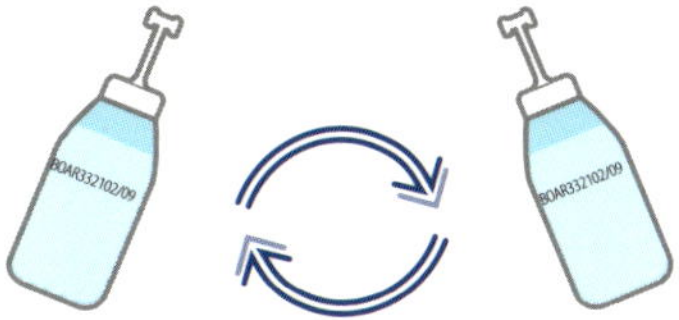

Figure 2. Rotation of the dose to mix.

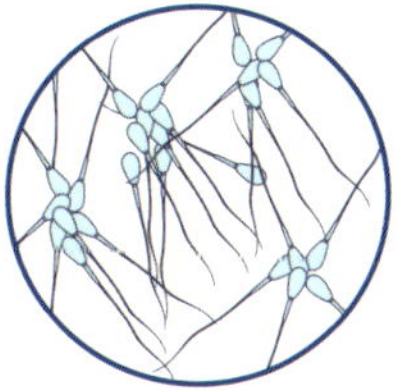

Figure 3. Clumped sperm.

Table 1. Types of movement of individual sperm.

Score and appearance	Name		The sperm...
0 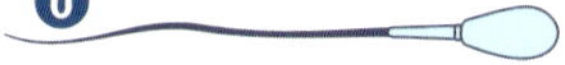	Akinesia		...does not move.
1 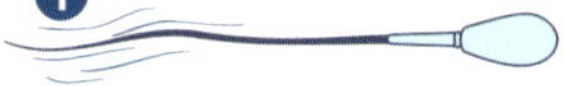	Oscillating and vibrating		...rotates but without progressive movement. The head stays still and the tail moves compulsively.
2 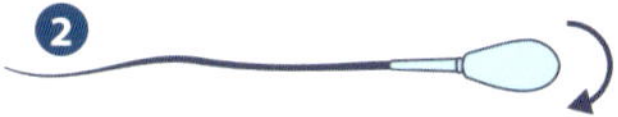	Circular		...moves in a circle of the same diameter as the length of the sperm.
3 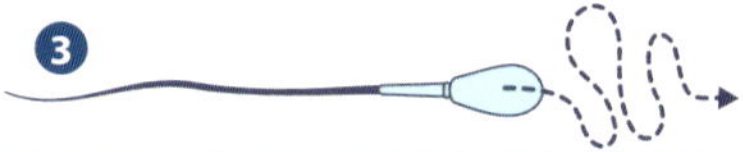	**Progressive** (the sperm generally advances, with progressive movements)	Sinuous	...tends to advance with sinuous movements.
4 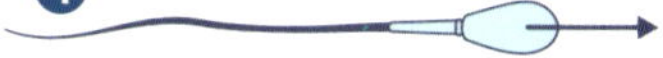		Rapid, in a straight line	...advances in a straight line and quickly.
5 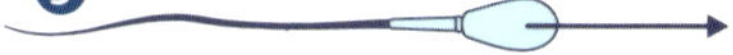		Very rapid, in a straight line	...advances in a straight line and very quickly.

To be suitable for insemination, over 70 % of the sperm sampled should display progressive movements. Even so, excellent sperm motility does not guarantee that the sperm are not damaged; without doubt, the more complete and technical the sperm assessment carried out by the artificial insemination centre (AIC), the better the quality of the sperm present in the semen doses.

If the semen dose is not suitable for artificial insemination, the reason for the failure in sperm motility should be determined, in the following order:

Farm

1. Check the temperature of the warming plate: 38 °C.
2. Repeat the study with a new drop of the same semen in case the observation period was excessively long.
3. Repeat the study with other semen doses, to see if other semen is affected.
4. Review the record of temperature fluctuations in the semen cooler, which should be kept at 15–17 °C during storage of the semen on the farm.
5. Check the records for semen temperature on arrival at the farm, together with the date and time.

→

AIC

6. Check the temperature records for the semen whilst in transit to the farm.
7. Check results for doses of the same ejaculate, retained for daily controls until the expiry date.
8. Ensure immediate dispatch of new semen doses to the farm.

Management of semen doses on the farm

The semen arrives on the farm diluted and packaged (Fig. 4) in a variety of bottles with screw or clip caps, tubes or bags, all clearly labelled with the number of the boar and the expiry date. The semen should immediately be stored in a semen storage unit and kept at a constant temperature of 15–17 °C.

Once the semen doses are removed from the cooler, they should be protected from ambient conditions that could damage the sperm, such as extremes of temperature, temperature changes, and excessive light. It is advisable to store the doses in a cool box or bag for protection until they are required for insemination.

Warming the semen in a water bath at 37 °C is recommended. However, it is better to inseminate at 15–17 °C if temperatures changes are expected during insemination.

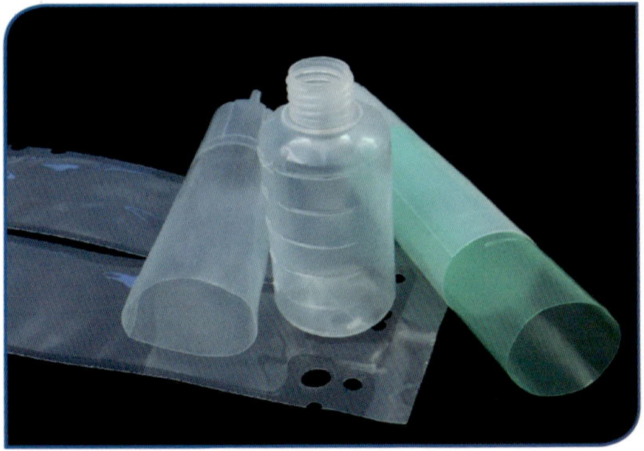

Figure 4. Different containers for pig semen doses.

Preparing the equipment required for artificial insemination

To avoid improvisation during insemination, ensure a standard procedure to prepare, organise and transport all materials in boxes or trolleys to the sows in oestrus in the farm insemination area.

The following equipment is required for insemination:

- Catheters.
- Gloves.
- Wipes moistened with a nonspermicidal disinfectant.
- Absorbent paper.
- Nonspermicidal lubricant.
- Marker or spray to mark each sow following insemination.
- Synthetic pheromones in a spray.
- Lumbar pressure equipment: belts, arches, harnesses, straps, saddlebags, etc. that stimulate the sow's lumbar area and prevent her from lying down during insemination. Some include weights (8–10 kg for gilts and 12–14 kg for adult sows) that imitate the weight of the boar.

Catheters

Catheters for artificial insemination in pigs are classified according to the location where they deposit the semen during insemination (Fig. 5).

Current catheter designs prevent injuries to the genital tract, as long as the sow is in oestrus when she is inseminated and the operator takes care.

Some gilts retain a vestige of a hymen at the junction of the vestibule and the vagina that might make it difficult to insert the catheter. Slight bleeding may occur when this is broken.

Once insemination is complete, any signs of blood on the catheter, or any other incidents, should be noted.

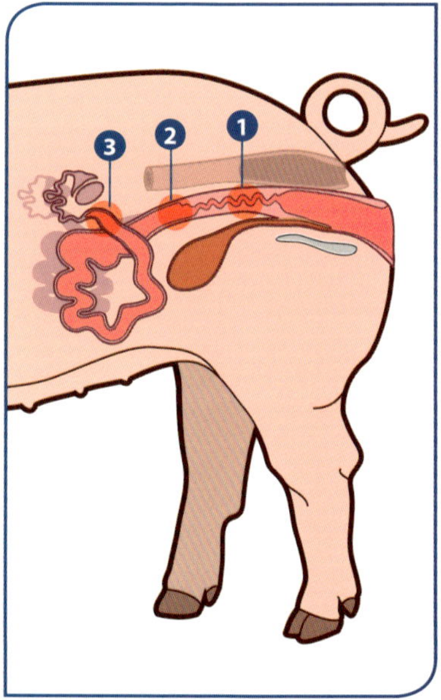

Figure 5. Locations where semen is deposited, according to the type of insemination. Cervix (1) for intracervical insemination, uterine body (2) for postcervical intrauterine insemination and uterine horn (3) for deep intrauterine insemination.

Common features of all AI techniques

Hygiene during AI

One overall and essential factor to prevent uterine diseases which cause reproductive failure is hygiene during the artificial insemination process. The cervix is open when the sow is in oestrus, to allow sperm to pass and, although the genital tract's defence mechanisms are heightened during this phase, bacteria could still enter the uterus.

It is essential to use a different catheter to inseminate each sow in order to eliminate any possibility of transmitting an infection from one female to another. These days, most farms use single-use disposable catheters. Catheters that are packaged individually provide the greatest level of hygiene during artificial insemination. The package is opened at the end with the insemination tip. As the catheter is gradually introduced into the vagina, the outer packaging is drawn backwards.

The deeper the proposed insemination, the more hygienic the insemination technique must be to prevent uterine infections and reproductive failure.

Introducing the catheter into the sow's vagina

The protocol employed by all artificial insemination techniques to introduce the catheter into the sow's vagina is as follows:

Step 1. When the sow is in oestrus, clean the vulva with a disposable wipe moistened with a **nonspermicidal** disinfectant and dry with a disposable paper towel.

Step 2. Lubricate the tip of the catheter with 1–2 ml of a **sterile, nonspermicidal** gel to facilitate introduction and prevent the catheter injuring the vaginal mucosa. Avoid plugging the catheter opening from where the semen will come out.

Step 3. Part the lips of the vulva and, while drawing them outwards, move the catheter towards the vaginal vestibule (Fig. 6).

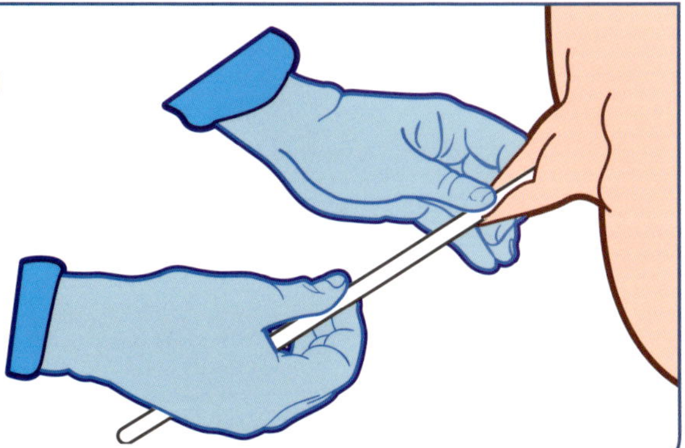

Figure 6. Opening the lips of the vulva and introducing the catheter.

Step 4. Gently introduce the catheter upwards towards the roof of the vagina at an angle of 45° to prevent damage to the external opening of the urethra (Fig. 7). If urine flows out of the free end of the catheter, it means that the catheter has been fed into the urethra. If this occurs, a new catheter should be used, as urine is spermicidal.

Step 5. Continue inserting the catheter in a more horizontal position.

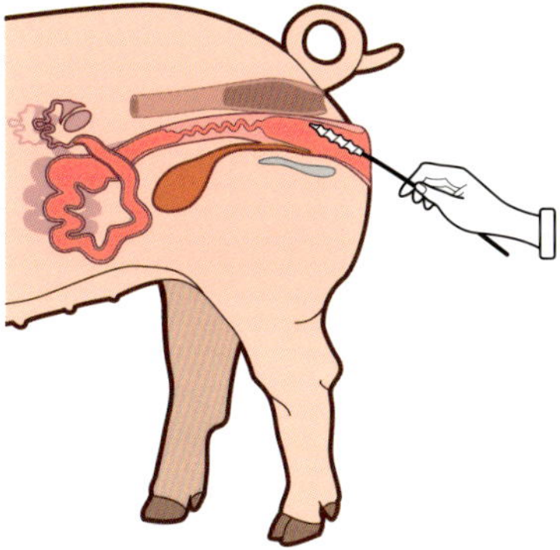

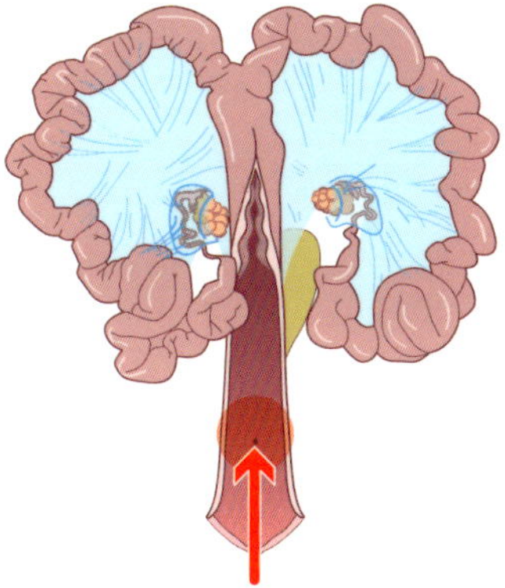

Figure 7. The catheter should be aimed at entry towards the roof of the vagina at an angle of 45°.

After this point, each insemination technique has its own peculiarities with regard to the part of the uterus where the semen is deposited: cervix, body or horn.

Intracervical insemination

The cervix has a wide vaginal part and another, narrower uterine area. Both have interdigitating pads that close the cervical canal like a zip (Fig. 8).

The intracervical insemination (IC-AI) technique, also called the classic, conventional or traditional technique, is the most similar to natural mating, in that the semen is deposited between the interdigitating pads of the vaginal region of the **cervix.**

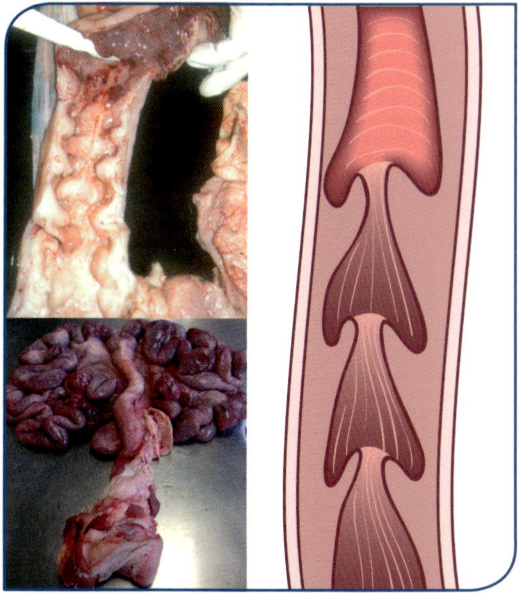

Figure 8. Interdigitating pads of the cervix in the sow. Catheters are designed to fit the pads in the same way as the boar's penis. Semen is deposited at the same site with intracervical insemination as with natural mating.

Catheters for IC-AI

The main differences between the various intracervical catheters on the market are the material they are made of and the shape of the insemination tip, which can be spiral-shaped (spirette-type) (Figs. 9a and b) or mushroom-shaped (Fig. 9c). The exterior end of the catheter can have an optional adaptor for the semen dose and a cap which prevents backflow. There are two sizes for use in gilts or sows.

There is also a system that combines the intracervical catheter and the semen dose in one piece (Fig. 9d). The vagina brings the semen up to temperature and the cervix melts the wax plug that prevents the semen from escaping during transport. The sow autoinseminates in approximately 10 minutes.

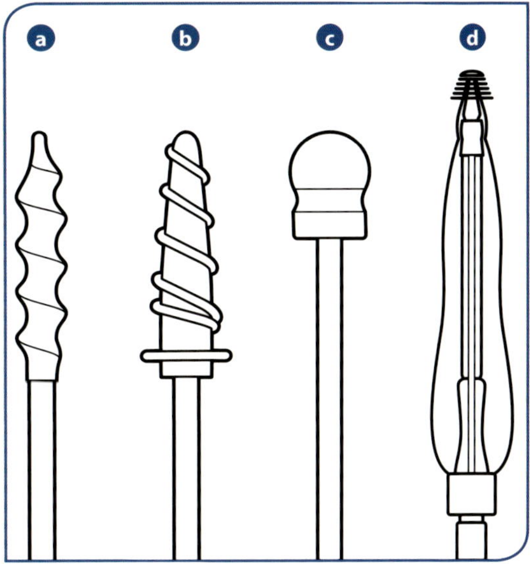

Figure 9. Catheters for intracervical artificial insemination.

IC-AI method

After introducing the catheter into the vagina, follow these steps:

1. There will be slight resistance to the catheter when it reaches the cervix.
   - If the catheter is the mushroom type, push forward until another resistance is felt.
   - If the catheter is the spirette type, rotate it in an anticlockwise direction.
2. Pull gently on the catheter to check that it is locked into the cervix.
3. Leave the intracervical catheter in position for 2–3 minutes before inseminating (while other receptive sows are inseminated).
4. Mix the semen dose gently and connect it to the free end of the intracervical catheter, and inseminate slowly (Fig. 10).
5. Remove the empty container, close off the catheter to prevent a backflow of semen and leave it in place for a few minutes to prolong mechanical stimulation of the cervix and encourage uterine contractions and passage of the sperm.
6. To remove the intracervical catheter, rotate it in a clockwise direction while pulling gently.

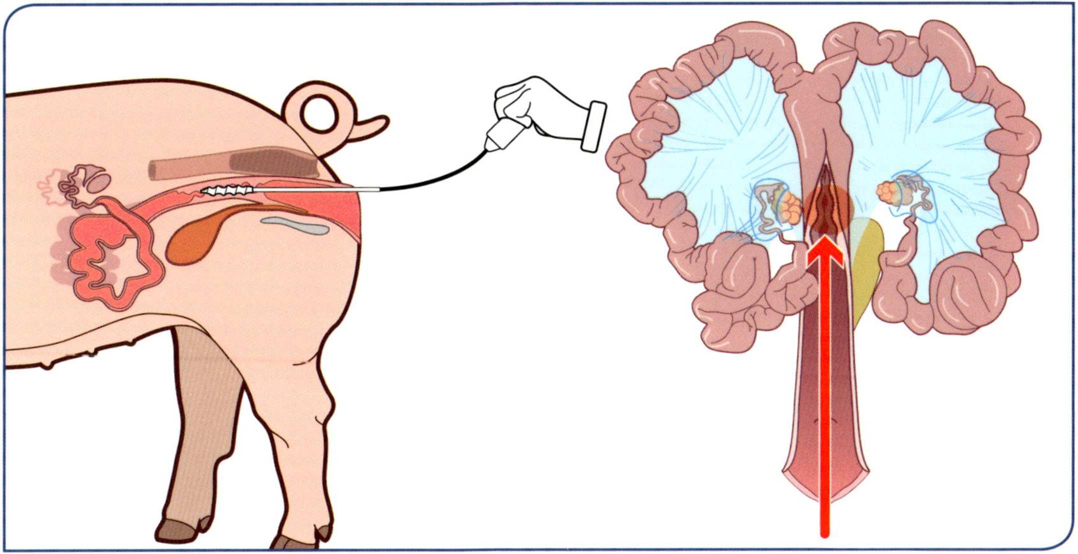

Figure 10. Intracervical artificial insemination.

Semen dose characteristics for IC-AI

A **volume of 80–100 ml** is required to enhance the passage of sperm from the cervix to the body of the uterus, and thus reduce loss by retention in the folds of the cervix or by backflow from the vulva. The **number of sperm** in the refrigerated dose should be high (**3,000 × 10^6**) because the distance to the oviduct is very long and many sperm will be phagocytosed by uterine defence mechanisms. If the semen is of an excellent quality, the AIC can reduce this to **2,200 × 10^6** sperm/dose; if frozen semen is used (which is rare), it should be increased to **6,000 × 10^6** sperm/dose.

Duration of intracervical insemination

The inseminator must be patient. It will take **3–8 min** to slowly introduce the semen dose and for it to be drawn up slowly by the sow towards the uterus, as it would be during natural mating.

Shorter times for IC-AI can affect the final fertility and prolificacy results.

Backflow from the vulva

In natural mating, the solids in the boar's semen form a plug in the cervix which prevents the backflow of semen. Intracervical catheters are designed to fit perfectly into the cervix and minimise the backflow of semen. Some have annular rings that form a seal and prevent backflow (Fig. 9b). Even so, it is common to see backflow from the vulva in the 4 hours following IC-AI.

When the loss is small and late, the backflow is considered to be physiological.

If the backflow is immediate and abundant, a large number of sperm can be lost and this can affect the sow's productivity. In this case, a note of this occurrence should be made in the sow's breeding records and she should be inseminated again.

The faster the insemination, the more likely there is to be semen backflow.

Stimulation of the sow during IC-AI

IC-AI is very laborious and requires an expert inseminator. The sow should be stimulated in the same way as she would be during natural mating:

- The presence of a boar (Fig. 11) and mechanical stimulation of the cervix with the insemination catheter to increase uterine contractions.
- Pressure on the back and massaging the flank, to increase the female's receptiveness.

There is a wide range of lumbar pressure equipment on the market and these also may hold the semen dose so that the sow absorbs the semen in time with the uterine contractions (**autoinsemination**), which reduces semen backflow. Such equipment enables the operator to inseminate several sows at once. In the absence of a boar, sow receptiveness can be increased by applying synthetic pheromones to the snout, but these do not have the same stimulatory effect on uterine contractions as being able to see the male. Uterine activity can be stimulated by applying a diluent warmed to 42 °C before insemination itself.

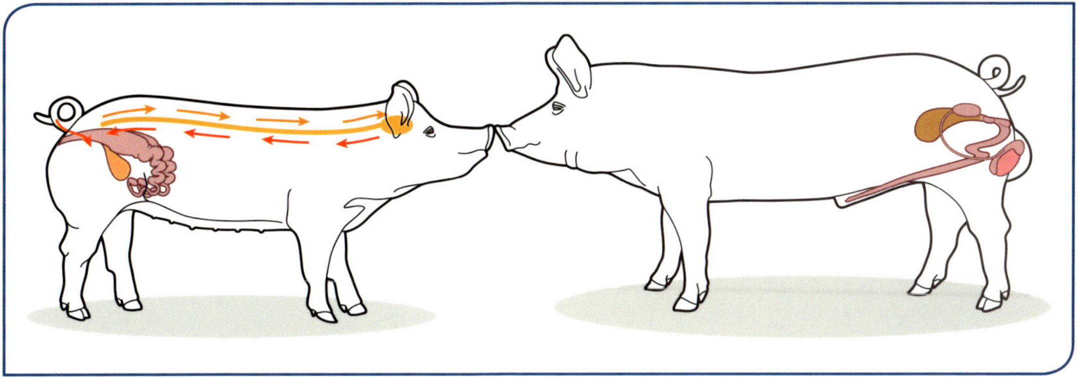

Figure 11. Using a boar to stimulate the sow.

Postcervical intrauterine insemination

When using the postcervical intrauterine artificial insemination (PC-AI) technique, semen is deposited in the uterine **body**.

Catheters for PC-AI

In PC-AI, the semen reaches the body of the uterus through a long, fine, and flexible catheter (Fig. 12). This is usually introduced as an inner catheter through the middle of an intracervical catheter that serves as a guide. The main differences between the different PC-AI inner catheters on the market are the material they are made of and their length and width, together with the location of the opening for the semen to exit into the uterus: frontal (with or without cap) or lateral. In some models, there are two sizes (for gilts and multiparous sows), as most catheters for multiparous sows are too big for gilts. There is a type of intracervical catheter that has an internal rubber membrane, which expands towards the uterine body as the semen enters the catheter.

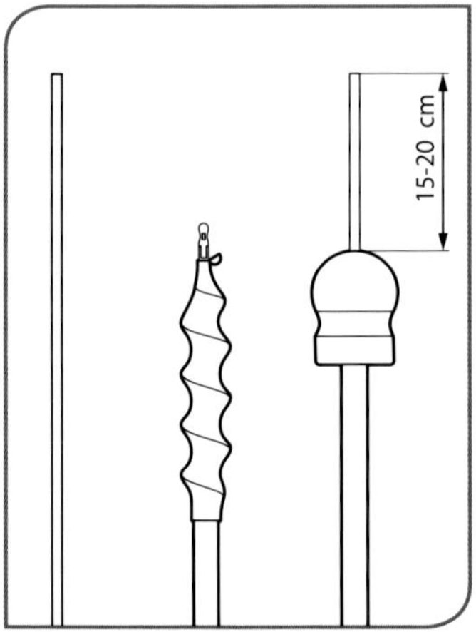

Figure 12. Catheters for postcervical intrauterine artificial insemination.

PC-AI method

The protocol for PC-AI is as follows:

1. If an intracervical catheter is used as a guide, wait 1–2 minutes for the cervix to relax.
2. Introduce the inner catheter and press forward sufficiently to overcome the resistance of the interdigitating pads of the cervix until the uterine body is reached (Fig. 13).
3. Squeeze to apply the semen dose in one go.
4. Once insemination is complete, twist the intracervical guide catheter several times to activate mechanical stimulation of the cervix and encourage uterine contractions and passage of the sperm.
5. Remove the intracervical guide catheter and the inner catheter as one piece.

If the inner catheter cannot initially be advanced, postpone insemination and try advancing again after some time has elapsed to allow the cervix to relax. If the inner catheter still cannot be fully advanced into the uterine body, do not persist with PC-AI. In this case, use IC-AI.

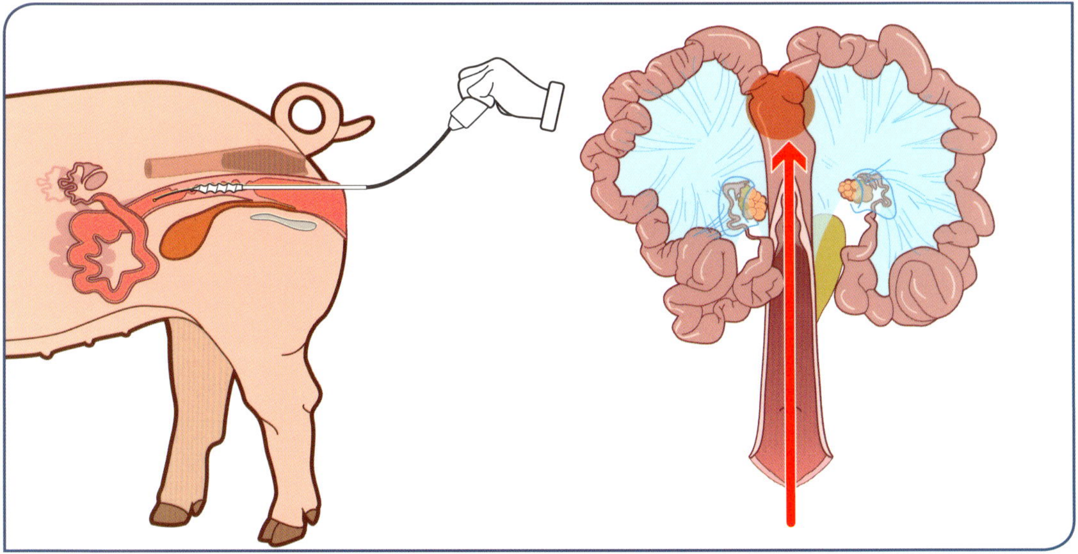

Figure 13. Postcervical intrauterine insemination.

Semen dose characteristics for PC-AI

As the semen is deposited directly into the uterine body, the **volume** required for insemination is less than that needed in IC-AI, although **40–50 ml** is still required to accelerate the transport of the sperm to the distal extremity of the uterine horns.

The distance the sperm have to travel to the oviduct is shorter than in natural mating or IC-AI, so the **number of sperm** used in refrigerated doses can be less in PC-AI (**1,500 × 10^6**). If the semen is of an excellent quality, the AIC may reduce this to **750–1,000 × 10^6** sperm/dose. If frozen semen is used, the concentration should be greater than **2,500 × 10^6** sperm/dose.

Fewer sperm are used in this technique as there is no sperm retention in the cervix, losses through backflow at the vulva are minimal and virtually the only losses are caused by uterine defence mechanisms.

Advantages of PC-AI

- It is very quick and simple for the operator. After the inner catheter is placed in the uterine body, only about 1 minute is needed to squeeze the semen directly into the uterus. The time saved can be used for other farm work.
- It does not require the presence of a boar, or stimulation of the sow. The cervix must be very relaxed for the inner catheter to pass easily through the interdigitating pads to the uterine body.
- The reduced numbers of sperm required per dose for PC-AI increases the productivity of AI centres' high genetic value boars.
- More sows can be inseminated with semen from the same boar, so more homogeneous piglets can be produced on the farm.
- Despite its advantages, the fertility and prolificacy results are not statistically significantly different from those obtained by intracervical insemination.
- PC-AI is compatible with a single insemination at a fixed interval after hormonal induction of ovulation, and also with insemination with good quality frozen-thawed semen.

Deep intrauterine insemination

Deep intrauterine artificial insemination (DIU-AI) consists in depositing semen at the end of a uterine **horn.** It is not commonly used on-farm.

Catheters for DIU–AI

In DIU–AI, semen is deposited at **the distal end of one of the uterine horns,** near the oviduct, through a very long, flexible catheter (over 1.5 m long) that is introduced through the middle of an intracervical catheter that acts as a guide (Fig. 14). Sterility of the catheter is maintained throughout the whole insemination process, as it is protected in plastic sleeves. One model additionally deposits some of the semen in the cervix.

One type of catheter has been designed for the nonsurgical transfer of embryos and this, along with new embryo storage techniques, has enabled embryos to be transferred in specialist breeding units.

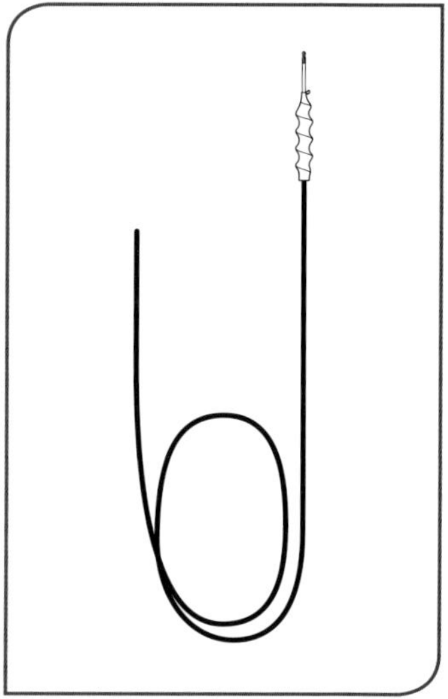

Figure 14. Long flexible catheter for DIU–AI.

DIU-AI method

The protocol for DIU-AI is as follows:

1. After the intracervical guide catheter is inserted, wait a few minutes for the cervix to relax.
2. Introduce the inner catheter and press forward sufficiently to overcome the resistance of the interdigitating pads of the cervix until the uterine body is reached.
3. Continue to press forward, and it will pass into one of the uterine horns.
4. Continue to press very slowly to introduce the full length of the catheter into the uterine horn.
5. Introduce the semen dose in one go (Fig. 15).
6. Once insemination is complete, remove the deep intrauterine (inner) catheter very slowly. Then twist the intracervical catheter several times to activate mechanical stimulation of the cervix and encourage uterine contractions and passage of the sperm.
7. Remove the intracervical guide catheter.

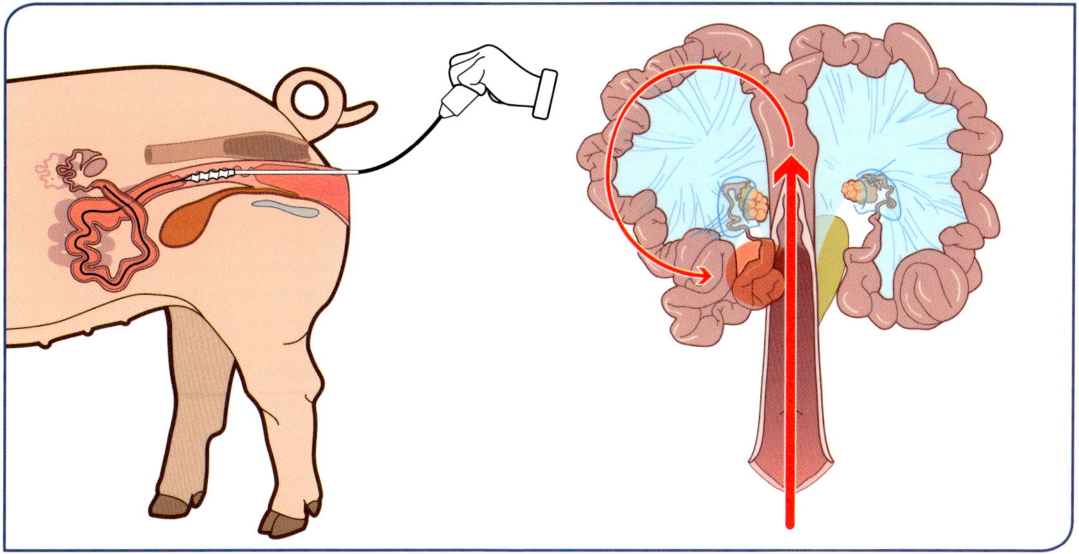

Figure 15. Deep intrauterine insemination.

Semen dose characteristics for DIU-AI

The distance the sperm have to travel from the end of the uterine horn to the oviduct is minimal, so the **volume (20 ml)** and the **number of sperm** used in refrigerated doses can be very low (**600×10^6**), as there are no losses from the vulva due to backflow, or retention in the cervix, and uterine phagocytosis is minimal. If the semen is frozen, the concentration should be greater (**$1{,}000–1{,}500 \times 10^6$**).

Advantages and disadvantages

- Although DIU-AI does not require the presence of a boar or stimulation of the sow, it is more laborious than PC-AI, takes a little longer to carry out and requires previous operator training. The special features of the catheter make it expensive.
- Frozen semen is suitable for use in DIU-AI in breeding programmes. The poorer the quality of the frozen-thawed semen used, the closer to the oviduct it should be deposited.

The deeper the insemination point, the fewer sperm are required for fertilisation in the oviduct, so this technique is essential when there are only a small number of spermatozoa, such as with sexed semen.

Use of seminal additives during artificial insemination

The boar's seminal plasma becomes very diluted in artificial insemination, so semen doses have hardly any of the substances and hormones that would stimulate uterine contractions and participate in the process of ovulation in natural mating. One strategy to improve fertility and prolificacy (especially during the summer) is to add various substances to the refrigerated or frozen semen dose at the time of insemination. These additives can include hormones, enzymes, and sperm motility stimulants.

A system of semen photoactivation may improve semen quality and, therefore, the farm's breeding results.

For breeding sows, hormonal control and farming methods (weaning, boar effect, flush feeding, etc.) vary from farm to farm. The objective is for enough sows to be in oestrus at regular intervals to support an insemination programme and meet production targets.

When choosing the type of hormone to use for each sow, the date of the last event in the sow's breeding records should be taken into consideration (oestrus, insemination, abortion, farrowing, weaning, administration of other hormones, etc.). Diagnostic techniques, such as ultrasound and progesterone testing, are sometimes also required to ascertain the condition of the ovaries.

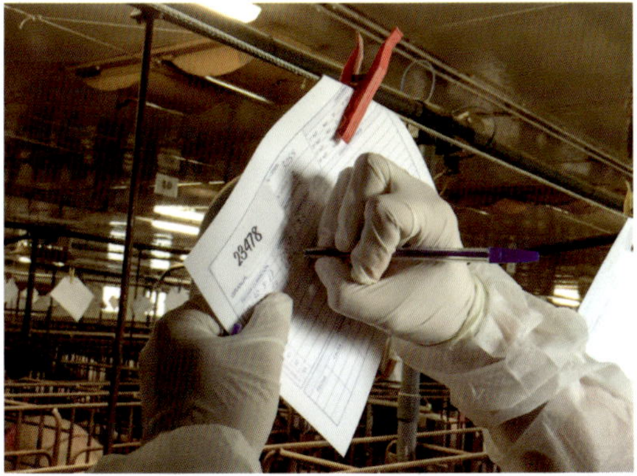

Figure 1. Recording data in the sow's breeding records.

Accurate and detailed breeding records must be kept for each sow to enable effective hormone control on the farm.

The **hormone options** usually available for use in pigs (check country-specific variations) are listed below.

- Gonadotropin-releasing hormone (GnRH) analogues:
  - Buserelin.
  - Gonadorelin.
  - Peforelin.
- Gonadotropins:
  - Equine chorionic gonadotropin (eCG).
  - Human chorionic gonadotropin (hCG).
- Progestogens: altrenogest.
- Prostaglandins:
  - PGF2α.
  - Prostaglandin analogues: alphaprostol and cloprostenol.

Less frequently used alternatives are porcine LH, goserelin, lecirelin, and triptorelin.

Hormone treatments to control oestrus on pig farms are used for:

1. Induction of oestrus.
2. Synchronisation of oestrus.
3. Combined induction and synchronisation of ovulation during oestrus.

Detailed knowledge of the reproductive physiology of the sow during the oestrous cycle and the pharmacology of the various reproductive hormones is essential to design an effective hormone programme.

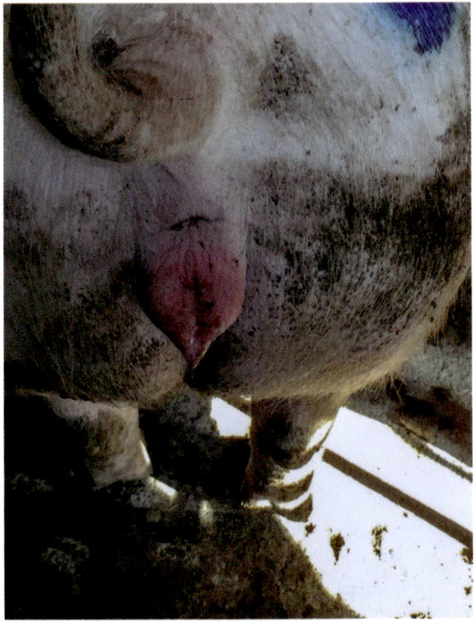

Figure 2. Vulva of a sow in oestrus.

Hormones can only be prescribed by a veterinary practitioner. Data sheets with comprehensive and updated information are available for each product from the EMA (European Medicines Agency) online information centre.

EMA data sheets (http://www.ema.europa.eu/ema/)

- Indications for treatment.
- Dosage.
- Route of administration.
- Contraindications.
- Adverse effects.
- Precautions for use.
- Interactions with other medication.
- Storage conditions.
- Withdrawal period before slaughter, etc.

Hormones should only be used on the farm under veterinary supervision. All hormones should be handled with gloves to prevent potential absorption by the skin.

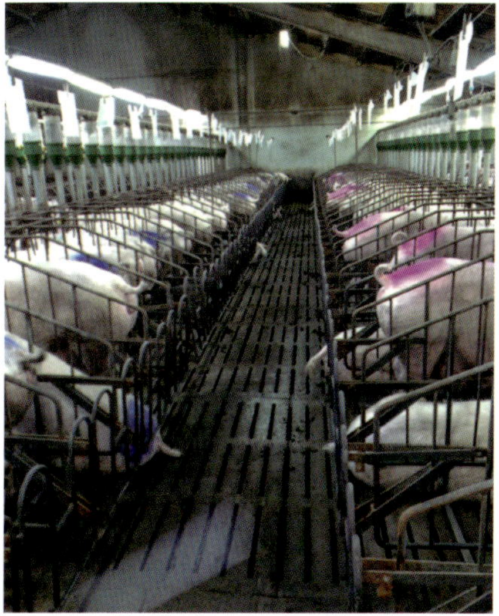

Figure 3. Insemination area on a commercial farm.

Induction of oestrus

First oestrus occurs in young gilts when they reach **puberty** at 6–7 months of age. **Weaning the piglets** and the **presence of a boar** tend to be enough of a stimulus to bring breeding sows into oestrus in the first week after weaning. If a sow fails to come into oestrus, she is said to be in **anoestrus,** as her hypothalamic–pituitary–ovarian axis is not functioning and is unable to induce oestrus and ovulation.

It is advisable to select sows that come into oestrus easily as breeding stock. However, it may be necessary to **use hormones to stimulate the ovaries** of **anoestrous sows** to bring enough animals into oestrus to carry out the scheduled number of inseminations. This is common practice in summer, due to the seasonal nature of reproduction in the sow.

Hormone treatments should never replace good breeding management. If more than 7–10 % of sows on the farm are in anoestrus, the causes must be ascertained and corrected.

Of the sows sent for slaughter because they were supposed to be in anoestrus, 40 % actually have ovaries that have ovulated recently and cyclic hypothalamic–pituitary–ovarian axes. These sows have been wrongly classified as nonovulatory, and thus in anoestrus, but are actually in **pseudoanoestrus**, as this condition is termed. This misclassification is usually due to a failure to detect oestrus. Table 1 shows the causes of absence of oestrus in the sow.

Table 1. Causes of absence of oestrus (Falceto, 2015).

Physiological anoestrus	Anoestrus	Pseudoanoestrus	Ovarian disease
• Not yet reached puberty. • Gestation. • Lactation. • 7–10 days postweaning.	• Delayed puberty (>8 months). • Noncyclic after first oestrus. • Barren sow which has not come into oestrus. • >7–10 days after weaning.	• Silent oestrus (suboestrus). • Undetected oestrus (breeding and farrowing rooms). • Barren sow with undetected oestrus (gestation room). • Pregnant sow recorded as barren.	• Congenital. • Luteal cysts. • Luteinised follicular cysts. • Persistent corpora lutea. • Luteoma

Differentiating between anoestrus and pseudoanoestrus

- **Abdominal ultrasound.** Failure to detect oestrus in a sow even though it did occur can be confirmed by the absence of corpora lutea in the ovaries and of follicles larger than 6 mm. Ovarian cysts can also be diagnosed using this technique.
- **Progesterone (P4) hormone levels.** Progesterone levels of less than 1 ng/ml in blood samples taken from sows every 7 days for 3 consecutive weeks can confirm anoestrus (Figs. 4 and 5).
- **Postmortem examination of the ovaries.** Anoestrus can be confirmed by examination of the ovaries from a group of sows slaughtered for apparently not coming into oestrus. This will give an indication of whether the methods of detection of oestrus used on the farm are adequate (Figs. 6 and 7).

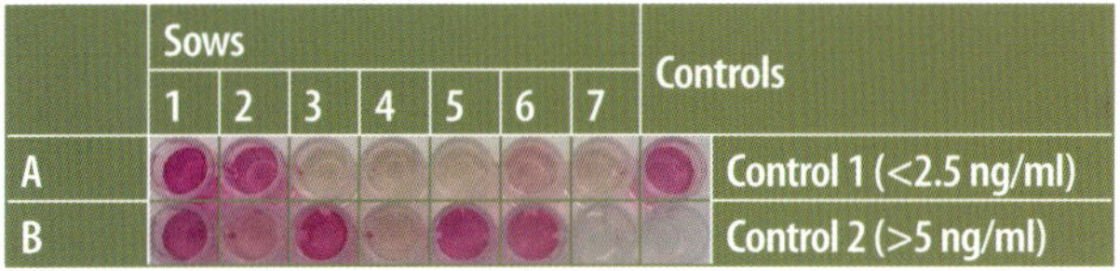

Figure 4. Rapid ELISA test for on-farm qualitative determination of progesterone in the blood.

The pink wells are consistent with basal levels of progesterone (control 1; <2.5 ng/ml), indicating sows that could be in anoestrus, and the transparent wells are consistent with high levels of progesterone (control 2; >5 ng/ml), indicating cyclic sows. The results of this test would be:

- Sows A1, A2, B1, B3, B5, and B6: progesterone levels <2.5 ng/ml (cyclic sows in pro-oestrus or oestrus, or noncycling sows, thus in anoestrus).
- Sows A3, A4, A5, A7, B4, and B7: progesterone levels >5 ng/ml (cyclic sows in the luteal phase, pregnant, or with luteal or luteinised cysts).
- Sows A6 and B2: progesterone levels between 2.5 and 5 ng/ml (cyclic sows that have just ovulated or are at the end of the luteal phase).

The exact levels of P4 in the blood should be ascertained by sending blood serum samples to a laboratory for analysis.

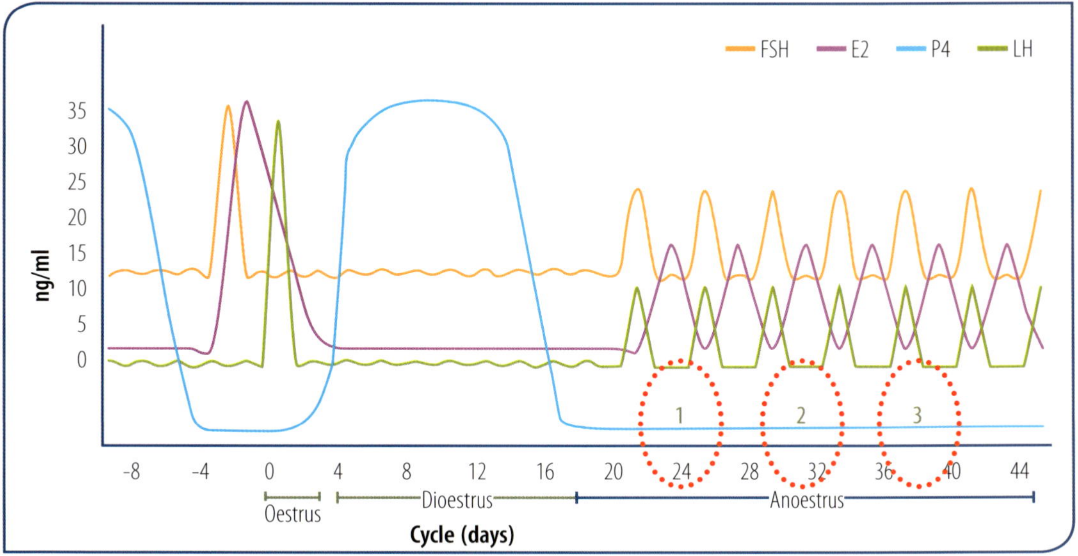

Figure 5. Sow in true anoestrus. Inactive ovary: P4 levels <1 ng/ml (1, 2 and 3). Treatment: gonadotropins for induction of oestrus. FSH: follicle-stimulating hormone; LH: luteinising hormone (Falceto, 2015).

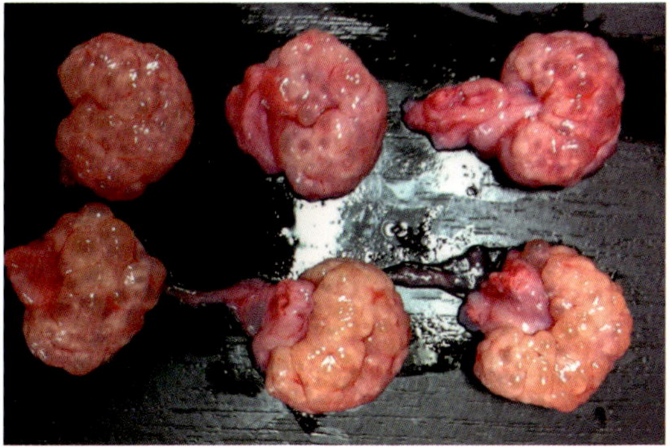

Figure 6. The ovaries of an anoestrous sow never have corpora lutea; these would indicate recent ovulation. They usually display some small and medium-sized follicles.

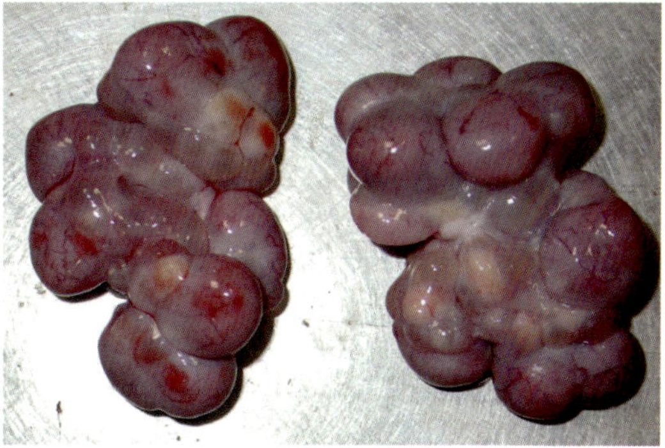

Figure 7. Corpora lutea in the ovaries indicate that the sow has ovulated recently and is cyclic (pseudoanoestrus).

Hormones that stimulate the ovaries

- **Gonadotropins**. The most common treatment for anoestrus is a combination of 400 IU of eCG and 200 IU of hCG administered intramuscularly (IM) or subcutaneously (SC) in the neck. In combination, they can induce oestrus 3–6 days after administration. In sows, they are administered on the day of weaning or 24 hours later. In gilts, they should be given immediately after progestogen withdrawal. This system can also prevent summer anoestrus, especially in gilts. Gonadotropins can also be used to induce early puberty in gilts over 140–150 days of age. Older and heavier prepubescent gilts come into oestrus better and subsequently also cycle better.
- **GnRH analogues (peforelin)**. These are injected IM 24 hours after weaning or 48 hours after progestogen withdrawal, to prevent summer anoestrus.

It is advisable to use hormonal induction of oestrus in combination with sexual stimulation of the sow by the presence of a boar.

Absence of oestrus after hormonal induction

- Disease.
- Poor body condition.
- Pseudoanoestrus: the ovaries are cyclic and oestrus occurs after dioestrus, and not after hormonal induction. Treatment with gonadotropins during dioestrus can cause ovarian cysts.
- Use of unsuitable hormones to treat anoestrus:
    - Prostaglandins: there are no corpora lutea to be luteolysed.
    - Progestogens: the sow is in anoestrus when they are administered, and she will remain in anoestrous after withdrawal.

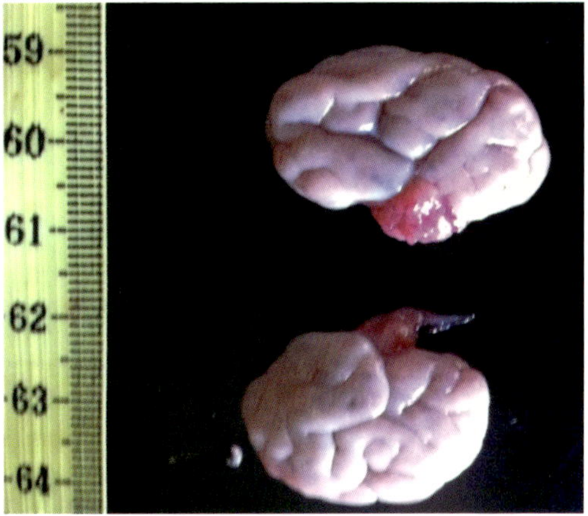

Figure 8. Ovaries in deep anoestrus. These hardly have even small follicles on the surface.

Synchronising oestrus

Weaning the piglets triggers oestrus after 3–7 days. However, for sows that are not postweaning, it is difficult for the farm to schedule sows for insemination, because it is not known when they will come into oestrus.

Replacement sows make up about 22 % of inseminations and it is very useful to synchronise them for insemination on a particular day.

Hormonal synchronisation of oestrus is used in gilts and unclassified sows (those returning to oestrus, postabortion, negative pregnancy diagnosis, etc.). Sows due to come into oestrus in the week they are scheduled to be inseminated (i.e. postweaners) do not need to be synchronised.

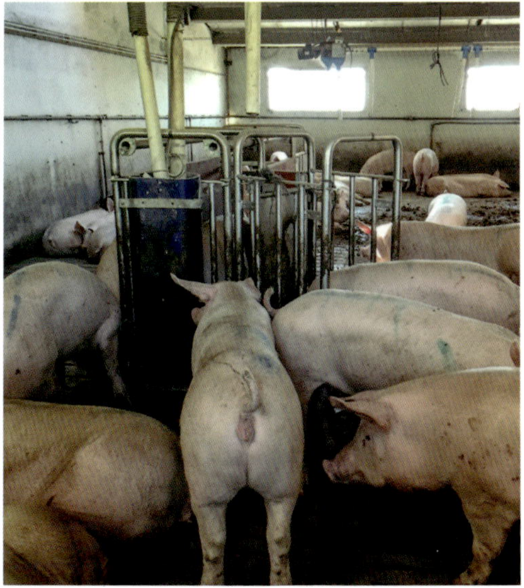

Figure 9. Group of replacement sows.

Hormones for synchronisation of oestrus

Synthetic progestogens are used to synchronise oestrus: **altrenogest** at 20 mg/sow/day is used in gilts and sows. It functions in a similar way to natural progesterone, blocking the hypothalamic–pituitary–ovarian axis, and therefore the development of oestrus. Its effects last while it is being administered orally, and oestrus occurs following withdrawal (2–3 days later in sows and 3–5 days later in gilts).

It is advisable to stimulate the gilt/sow with a boar after withdrawing altrenogest.

The withdrawal period for altrenogest is 24 hours before slaughter.

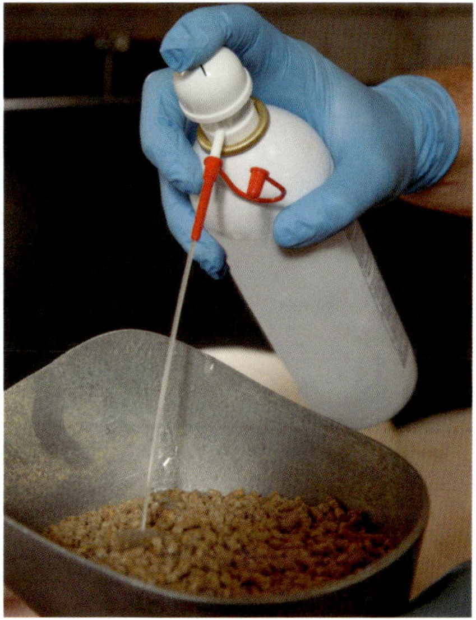

Figure 10. Dosing the feed with altrenogest.

Altrenogest is administered in the following ways on the farm:

- Mixed with a small amount of feed and given to each gilt/sow before the first feed each day.
- Directly into the mouth of each gilt/sow using a dosing gun.
- Using electronic automatic feeding stations designed for use with altrenogest, which is useful on very large farms. Altrenogest should be administered manually to gilts/sows that will not take it in their feed.

In order to synchronise oestrus effectively in sows and gilts that are to be inseminated at the same time, altrenogest treatment of the gilts should be stopped one day before the sows are weaned.

Gilts that are being synchronised with altrenogest should have already come into oestrus twice so that they can be inseminated the third time.

The gilts or sows must always be monitored to ensure that they consume their dose of altrenogest.

Absence of oestrus after synchronisation

Oestrus may not occur after hormonal synchronisation because:

- The product has not been administered correctly. Altrenogest must be administered at the same time each day, and the gilt/sow must consume the entire dose.
- No cycling. If the sow was not cyclic when the progestogen was administered, she is unlikely to be cyclic when it is withdrawn.

Progestogens should not be given to sows with a vaginal discharge, as they can exacerbate uterine infections.

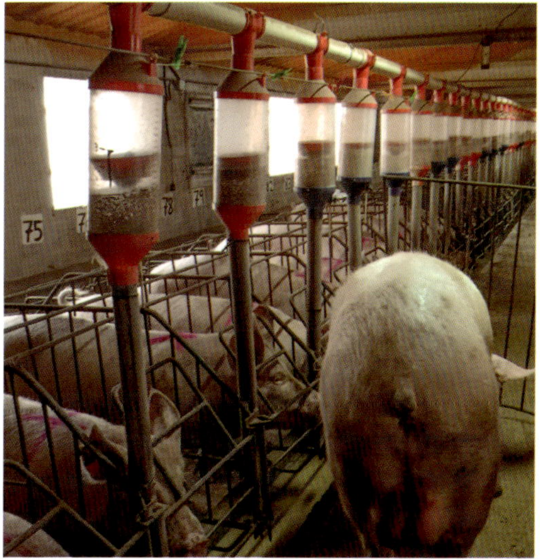

Figure 11. Cyclic sows come into oestrus after synchronisation with progestogens.

Duration of treatment

When the date of the previous oestrus is unknown

In this case, altrenogest should be administered for 18 days.

The corpora lutea last 16–18 days in dioestrus. Altrenogest blocks oestrus but does not affect luteolysis. Administered for at least 18 consecutive days, it ensures that no progesterone is produced that could block oestrus. When the progestogen is withdrawn, a new follicular phase starts, leading to oestrus.

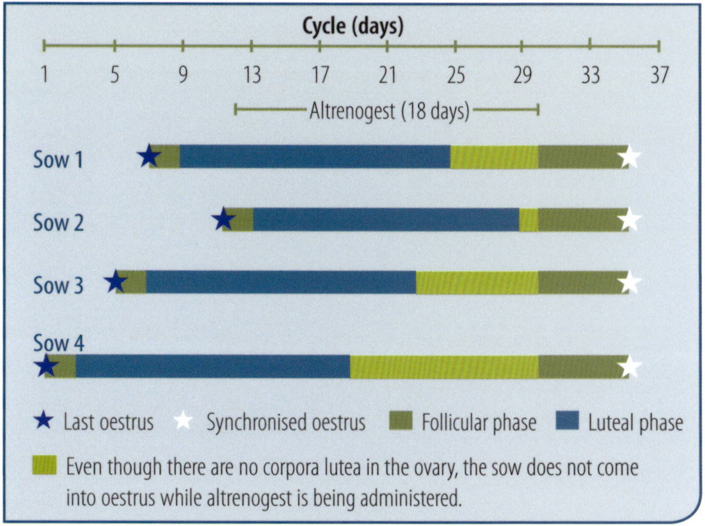

Figure 12. Administration of altrenogest for 18 consecutive days when the date of the previous cycle is unknown (Falceto, 2015).

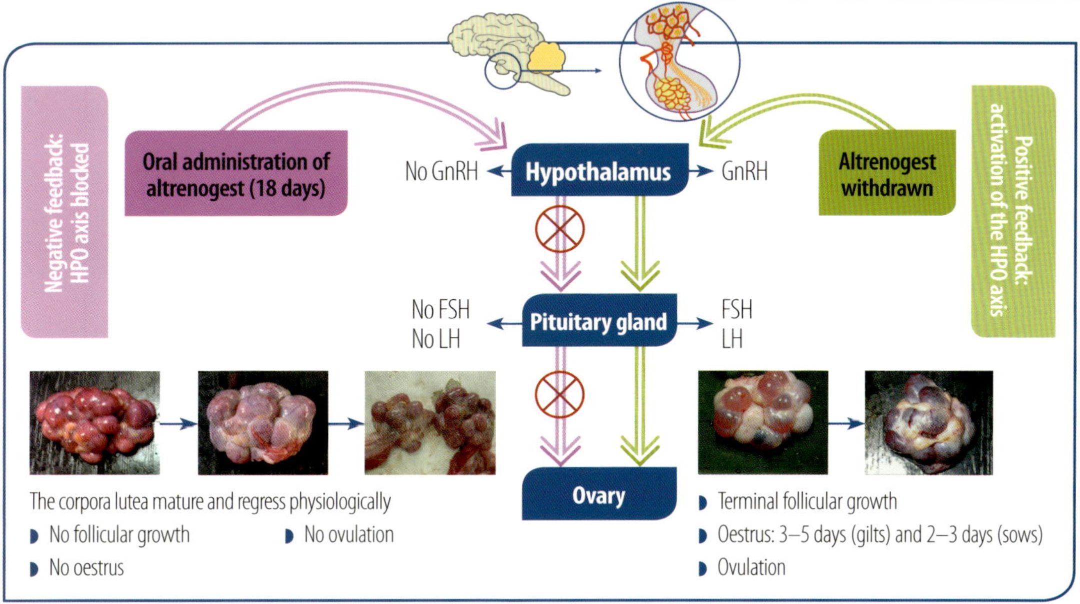

Figure 13. Hypothalamic–pituitary–ovarian (HPO) axis blocked after altrenogest administration. Activated after withdrawal.

When the date of the previous oestrus is known

If the date of the previous oestrus is known, the number of days that altrenogest is administered before insemination can be reduced. The duration of treatment with altrenogest is calculated by subtracting the number of days since the sow's last oestrus from the 18 days' duration of the luteal phase, as it is unlikely that any corpora lutea will remain in the ovary after that, and there will therefore be no progesterone to block oestrus.

Altrenogest should not be administered to gilts or sows showing signs of oestrus because it could cause ovarian cysts.

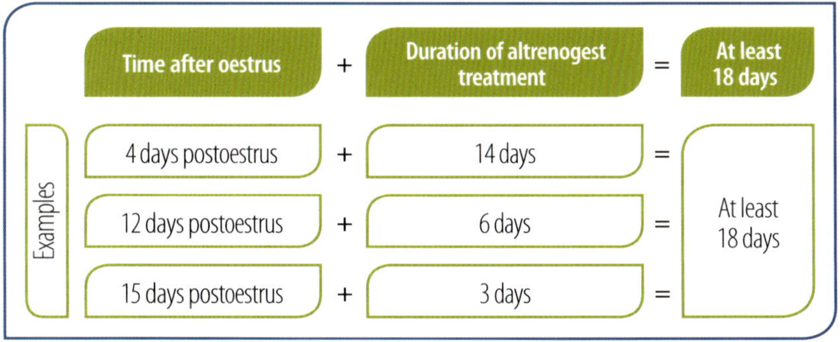

Figure 14. Altrenogest administration when the date of the previous oestrus is known.

Other uses for altrenogest on the farm

- **At weaning**. Progestogens are useful in **very thin** sows where it is desirable to delay oestrus, especially during periods of seasonal infertility. This situation is common after **lactations of less than 21 days** and at weaning in **primiparous sows** that are still growing during lactation. In order to recover body condition before the next oestrus, altrenogest is used for 8 days, starting on the day before weaning. Treated sows come into oestrus 4–5 days after altrenogest is withdrawn and they are inseminated at the same time as the sows weaned in the following week.

- **During lactation when there is spontaneous oestrus**. The objective is to synchronise the sows so that they come into oestrus in the first week after weaning. Altrenogest is administered from day 14 postfarrowing until the day that the piglets are weaned. The sows come into oestrus 4–5 days after altrenogest is withdrawn, and they are inseminated in the same way as any other weaned sow. The cause of this oestrus should be investigated whilst altrenogest is administered.

Induction and synchronisation of ovulation

The duration of oestrus and the timing of ovulation are very variable. However, when ovulation is induced hormonally, duration and timing can be synchronised and all **inseminations can be scheduled to a fixed timetable**.

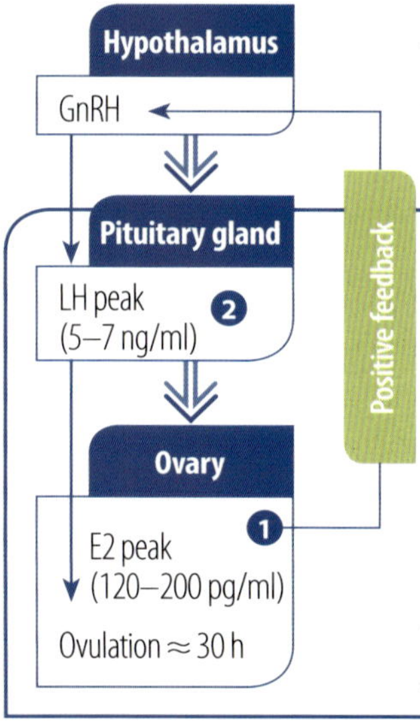

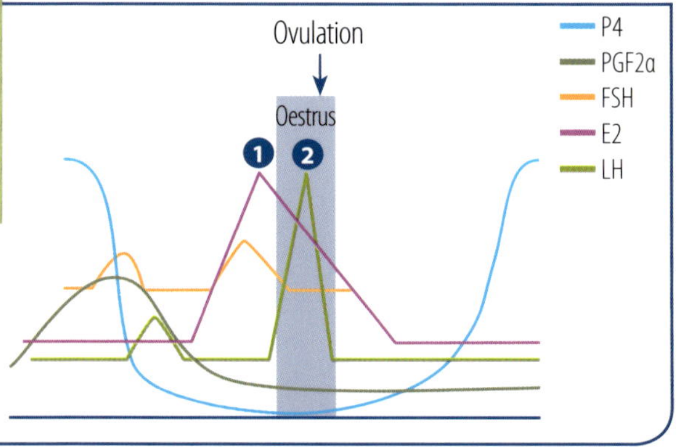

Figure 15. Diagram of the hormone cycle and ovulation in the sow.

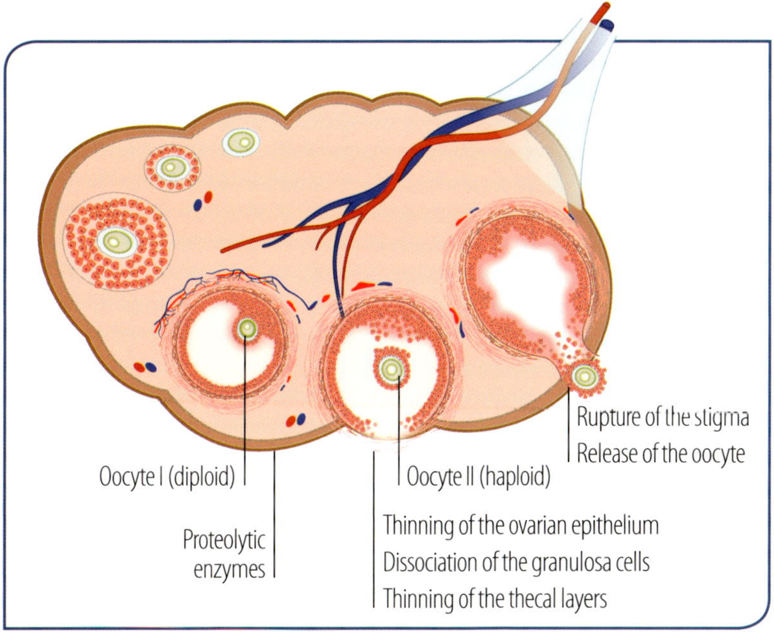

Ovulation is caused by the LH peak that follows maximum oestrogen concentration, which is mediated by GnRH.

GnRH analogues can induce an LH peak of a similar size to that produced by GnRH, and cause ovulation.

Figure 16. Ovary and ovulation.

When to induce ovulation during the oestrous cycle

Ovulation can only be induced in a sow in **pro-oestrus** after weaning or altrenogest treatment. The ovary will be in the terminal follicular phase with mature follicles that can respond to the luteinising hormone (LH) peak induced by the hormone treatment.

Induction of ovulation will fail in gilts or sows that are not in pro-oestrus (prepubescent gilts synchronised with altrenogest, sows in postweaning anoestrus or dioestrus following an undetected oestrus when lactating).

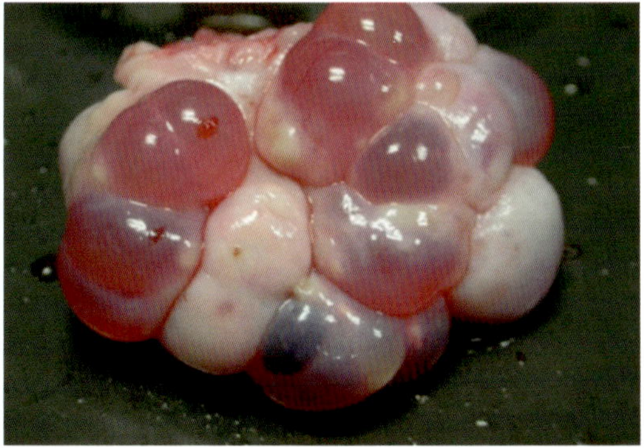

Figure 17. Ovary in pro-oestrus.

Hormones for induction of ovulation

GnRH analogues:

- The procedure used to synchronise ovulation with **gonadorelin** (IM/SC) always requires pro-oestrus to be guaranteed, by administering peforelin or eCG after weaning or progestogen treatment. Sows are artificially inseminated twice immediately after this administration.
- **Buserelin** (IM/SC), however, is administered directly after weaning or progestogen treatment. Sows are artificially inseminated once 30–33 hours later. In summer, a combination of 400 IU eCG and 200 IU hCG can be administered before buserelin.
- **Triptorelin** is administered vaginally on the fourth day after weaning. Sows are artificially inseminated once 22 hours later.

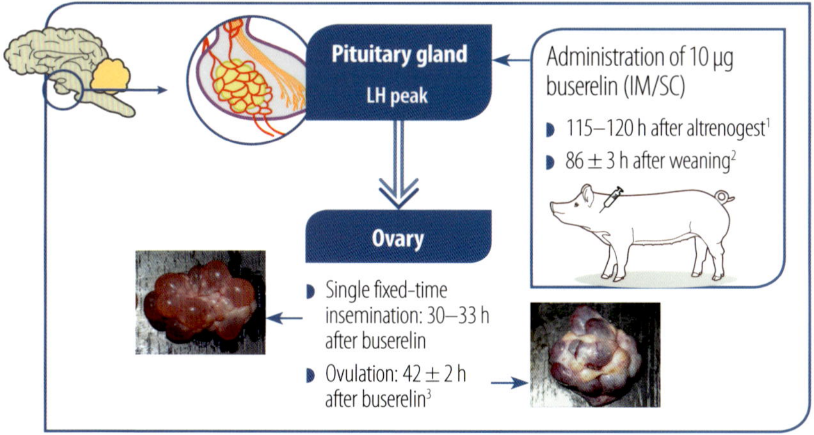

Figure 18. Hormonal induction of ovulation using buserelin.
[1]Driancourt, 2013.
[2]Martinat Botte et al., 2010.
[3]Van Kaufmann and Holtz, 1982.

It is still advisable to tease the sow to make sure that she is in oestrus before insemination, even though it is not strictly necessary.

GnRH analogues will fail to induce ovulation if the timetables for hormone administration and insemination are not adhered to.

Advantages of a single fixed-time insemination

- The weekly workload can be organised more effectively when the day and time at which all the sows should be inseminated is known. This also reduces the staffing levels required.
- Using a single semen dose per sow in oestrus allows all the sows in a group to be inseminated with semen from the same boar, reducing birth weight variability between litters.
- When ovulation and insemination are synchronised, fertilisation is also synchronised and farrowing is grouped more closely. Piglet birth weight is also more uniform across the same litter.
- Despite only inseminating each sow once, fertility and prolificacy reach similar levels to those obtained with multiple inseminations (Falceto et al., 2014).
- Inseminating more sows with semen from the same boar enables progeny to be evaluated sooner and genetics to be improved more rapidly.

References

DRIANCOURT MA, COX P, RUBION S, HARNOIS-MILON G, KEMP B, SOEDE NM. 2013. Induction of an LH surge and ovulation by buserelin (as Receptal) allows breeding of weaned sows with a single fixed-time insemination. *Theriogenology* 80(4):391–399.

FALCETO MV, ÚBEDA JL, CALAVIA M, GÓMEZ AB, COLLELL M, JIMÉNEZ M, MENJÓN R. 2014. Single fixed time insemination in multiparous sows with an injection of gonadotropin-releasing hormone agonist (Receptal). *6th European Symposium of Porcine Health Management,* Sorrento, Italy, Cod. 1501.

FALCETO MV. 2015. *Guías prácticas en producción porcina. Fisiopatología ovárica en la cerda.* 1st ed. Editorial Servet.

VON KAUFMANN F, HOLTZ W. 1982. Induction of ovulation in gonadotropin treated gilts with synthetic gonadotropin releasing hormone. *Theriogenology* 17(2):141–57.

KIRKWOOD RN, KAUFFOLD J. 2015. Advances in breeding management and use of ovulation induction for fixed-time AI. *Reproduction in Domestic Animals* 50 (Suppl. 2):85–89. doi: 10.1111/rda.12524. ISSN 0936-6768.

MARTINAT-BOTTE F, VENTURI E, GUILLOUET P, DRIANCOURT MA, TERQUI M. 2010. Induction and synchronization of ovulations of nulliparous and multiparous sows with an injection of gonadotropin-releasing hormone agonist (Receptal). *Theriogenology* 73:332–342.

ROCA J, PARRILLA I, BOLARIN A, MARTINEZ EA, RODRIGUEZ-MARTINEZ H. 2016. Will AI in pigs become more efficient? *Theriogenology* 86(1):187–93.

SÁNCHEZ-SÁNCHEZ R, MORELL J, LLAMAS PJ, GONZÁLEZ A, DE LA CRUZ P, MARTÍN LLUCH M, CARRASCOSA C, GÓMEZ FIDALGO E. 2014. Encapsulación seminal de semen de verraco (II). Resultados obtenidos en conservación seminal, transporte espermático y pruebas de inseminación. *Avances en Tecnología Porcina* 11(108): 52–58.

LIST OF ABBREVIATIONS

EMA: European Medicines Agency

CASA: computer-assisted sperm analysis

AIC: artificial insemination centre

E2: total oestrogens

eCG: equine chorionic gonadotropin

FSH: follicle-stimulating hormone

GnRH: gonadotropin-releasing hormone

hCG: human chorionic gonadotropin

AI: artificial insemination

IC-AI: intracervical artificial insemination

PC-AI: postcervical intrauterine artificial insemination

DIU-AI: deep intrauterine artificial insemination

WOI: weaning-to-oestrus interval

LH: luteinising hormone

P4: progesterone

PGF2α: prostaglandin F2α

HPO: hypothalamic–pituitary–ovarian axis

IM: intramuscular

SC: subcutaneous